DIABETIC-FRIENDLY RECIPES

Discover The Easiest And Most Delicious Recipes For
People With Type 1 And Type 2 Diabetes

BARBARA HAMMOND

original author of this work can be in any fashion deemed liable for any hardship or damages that may befall them after undertaking information described herein.

Additionally, the information in the following pages is intended only for informational purposes and should thus be thought of as universal. As befitting its nature, it is presented without assurance regarding its prolonged validity or interim quality. Trademarks that are mentioned are done without written consent and can in no way be considered an endorsement from the trademark holder.

TABLE OF CONTENTS

DIABETIC FRUIT BARS

1 c. chopped dates

1/2 chopped dried apricots 1/2 c. walnuts

1 1/2 tsp. baking powder 1/2 c. butter

1   1/3 c. rolled oats 1/4 c. oil

2   eggs

1 tsp. vanilla

1 c. flour

1 tsp. cinnamon

In saucepan, melt oil and butter, add dates and apricots. Remove from heat and beat in egg and vanilla. Combine dry ingredients and mix with rest of mixture. Bake in 9 x 13 inch pan for 20 minutes at 350 degrees.

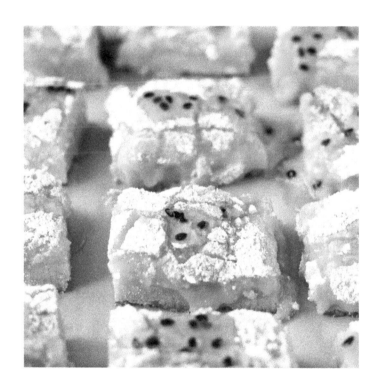

SMAKEROON COOKIES

3 egg whites

1/2 tsp. cream of tartar 2 tsp. sugar substitute 1/4 tsp. almond flavoring 3 c. Rice Krispies

1/4 c. shredded coconut

Beat egg whites until foamy, add cream of tartar and continue beating until stiff but not dry. Add sugar substitute and flavoring. Beat until blended. Fold in cereal and coconut and drop by teaspoonfuls onto lightly greased cookie sheet. Bake at 350 degrees for 12 15 minutes or until lightly browned. 1 serving = 1 fruit exchange (3 cookies).

Yields 24 cookies.

CHOCOLATE CAKE

1/4 c. sifted all purpose flour 1 tsp. baking powder

1/4 tsp. salt 3 tbsp. cocoa

1/4 c. cold coffee

1 tbsp. sugar substitute 1 egg

1 tbsp. salad oil 1/4 c. cold water 1 tsp. vanilla

Sift flour, baking powder, soda, and salt together. Blend cocoa and coffee. Beat egg and all sugar substitute, water, salad oil, and vanilla and stir into dry ingredients, mixing only until smooth. Stir in cocoa and coffee mixture. Line one 8 inch round layer cake pan with wax paper and grease with 1/8 teaspoon butter. Pour batter into pan, cover pan with foil and place in shallow pan of water. Bake at 350 degrees for 25 minutes. Remove from pan onto cake rack and cool. Cut layer in half crosswise to make half of a two layer cake. One serving = 1 fruit and 1 fat exchange.

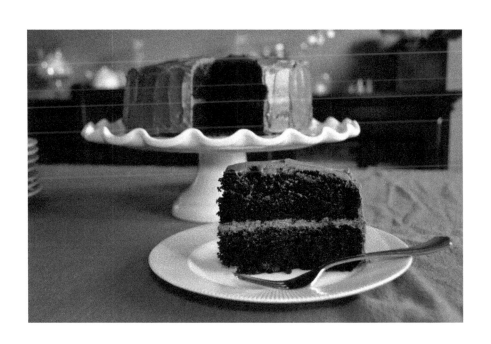

SPONGE CAKE

7 eggs

1/2 c. cold water

3 tbsp. sugar substitute 1/2 tsp. vanilla

2 tbsp. lemon juice

1/4 tsp. cream of tartar 1 1/2 c. cake flour

1/4 tsp. salt

Beat egg yolks until thick and lemon colored. Combine water, sugar substitute, vanilla, and lemon juice. Add to egg yolks beat until thick and foamy; add cream of tartar to beaten egg whites and continue beating until stiff peaks form. Fold carefully into yolk mixture. Combine sifted flour and salt. Sift a little at a time over the mixture, folding in gently. Pour into an ungreased 9 or 10 inch tube pan. Bake at 325 degrees for 1 hour and 15 minutes. One serving = 1 bread exchange.

CHOCOLATE SAUCE

1   tbsp. butter

2   tbsp. cocoa

1   tbsp. cornstarch 1 c. skim milk

2   tsp. sugar substitute 1/8 tsp. salt

Melt butter. Combine cocoa, cornstarch and salt; blend with melted butter until smooth. Add milk and sugar substitute and cook over moderate heat, stirring constantly until slightly thickened, remove from heat. Stir in vanilla. Set pan in ice water and stir until completely cold. (Sauce thickens as it cools.) One serving (1 tablespoon) free exchange.

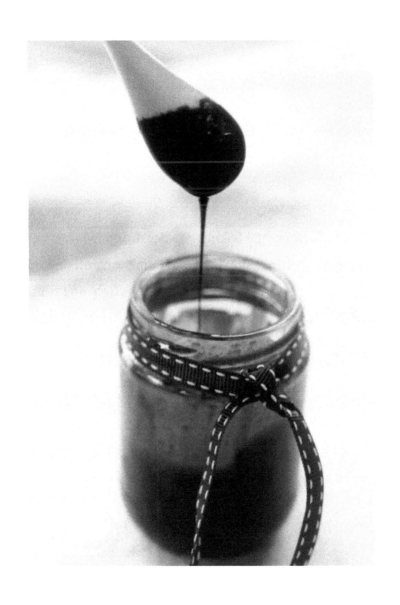

BUTTERSCOTCH COOKIES

1/2 tsp. baking powder 1 c. flour

 Pinch of salt

1/4 c. shortening

2 tbsp. brown sugar

1 env. or 1 1/16 oz. artificiallysweetened butterscotch pudding and pie filling mix

1/4 tsp. vanilla 1 egg

Sift together salt, flour, and baking powder. Combine shortening and sugar and cream together; slowly add pudding mix, mixing thoroughly. Then add egg, beat until mixture is light and fluffy. Stir in vanilla; and then add ingredients; mixing well. Place dough on wax paper; shape into a roll about 2 inches in diameter.

Wrap in wax paper. Place in freezer for about 30 minutes or refrigerate overnight. Cut into 1/8 inch slices then place on ungreased cookie sheet. Bake at 375 degrees for 8 10 minutes. 2 cookies = 2 fruit and 1 fat exchange. Makes 24 cookies.

MARASCHINO CHERRY - GUMDROP COOKIES

1/2 c. margarine 1/4 c. brown sugar 1 egg yolk

1 c. flour

1 1/2 tsp. vanilla extract 1/4 tsp. salt

24 sm. gum drops or 12 maraschino cherries, halved

Cream together margarine adding sugar slowly. Mix in egg yolk and vanilla extract. After sifting dry ingredients together slowly add creamed mixture. Roll into small balls and place on ungreased cookie sheet. Bake at 350 degrees for 5 minutes. After removing from oven, gently press maraschino cherry half or 1 gumdrop in the center of each cookie. Return to oven and continue baking for an additional 8 10 minutes. 2 cookies = 1 fruit exchange and 2 fat exchanges. Yields

2 dozen cookies.

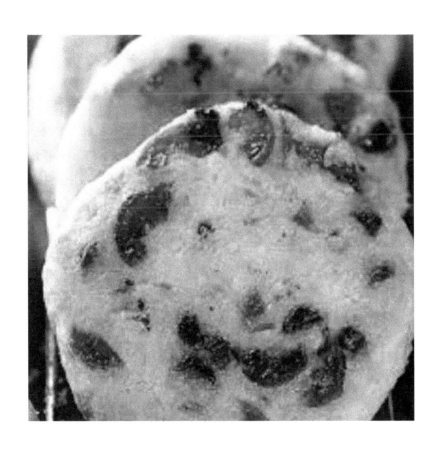

DIET 7 - UP SALAD

1 (4 serving) pkg. sugar free lemon gelatin 1 c. boiling water

6 oz. cold diet 7 Up

1 (8 oz.) (or 1/2 of 20 oz.) can drained crushed pineapple canned in its own juice (unsweetened)

1 banana, split and sliced

Dissolve gelatin in hot water. Set aside to cool slightly, then slowly add the chilled pop, pineapple, and banana pieces. Pour into an 8 inch square pan and chill until set. Add topping.

TOPPING

Cook over double boiler until thickened: 1 tbsp. flour Artificial Sweetener = 1/4 c. sugar 1/2 c. reserved juice 1 tbsp. low fat margarine Let cool, then fold in 1 envelope of prepared D Zerta whipped topping. Spread on top of the above "set" salad. 1 serving = 2 1/2 inch square; 1 fruit and 1 fat exchanges. Note: If this salad is doubled and a 9 x 13 inch pan is used, do not double the topping mixture. It's sufficient to cover all.

SAUCY CRANAPPLE SALAD

1 env. unflavored gelatin

1/4 c. cold water to soften above

1   (4 serving) pkg. sugar free raspberry gelatin 1 c. boiling water

2   c. (1/2 lb.) frozen cranberries

1 c. juice pack unsweetened crushed pineapple* with juice 1 c. unsweetened applesauce*

5 packets artificial sweetener

Place the clean, still frozen berries in the boiling water. Return to boiling and allow berries to pop open (8 to 15 minutes). Do not stir! Soften the unflavored gelatin in the 1/4 cup cold water, then add both gelatins to the hot cranberries; stir until dissolved. Add the pineapple with juice, the applesauce, and sweetener. Do not prepare this in a gelatin mold! Stir. Pour into a 10 cup mold and chill until set. 1 serving = 1 fruit exchange (approximately 60 calories).

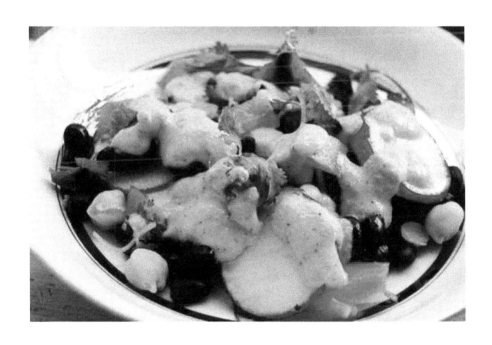

PINEAPPLE COLE SLAW

12 c. shredded cabbage (about 3 lbs.) 1 c. miniature marshmallows
2 lg. (20 oz.) cans prechilled* juice pack pineapple tidbits, drained

Toss with:DRESSING:

1/4 c. reserved pineapple juice Artificial sweetener = 1/4 c. sugar 1
1/2 c. lite Miracle Whip

Mix in a blender. Mix with slaw. Just before serving, add 2 split and
sliced bananas. The slices may be placed in enough pineapple juice
to cover; this will prevent them from turning brown until ready to
use. 1 serving = 3/4 cup: 1 veg, 3/4 fat, 1 fruit exch. About 105 cal.

DIETETIC PASTA SALAD

Corkscrew pasta

4 fresh mushrooms, sliced 1 cucumber, sliced

Kraft reduced calorie zesty Italian dressing 1 onion, sliced

1 tomato, diced

1 green pepper, chopped

Cook and rinse pasta in cold water. Mix with remaining ingredients and marinate in dressing. Chill and serve.

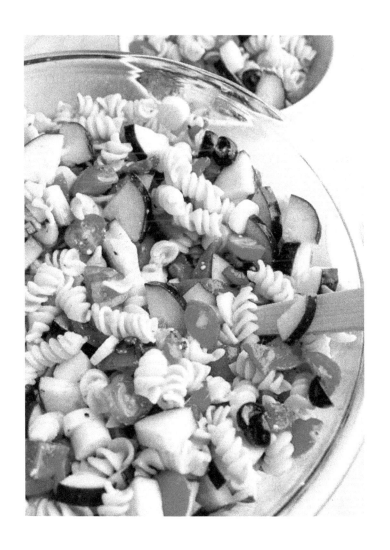

LASAGNA

1 c. chopped onions

1 c. sliced mushrooms

1/2 c. diced green peppers 1 tbsp. parsley flakes

1/2 tsp. each basil, oregano, chili powder 5 oz. Mozzarella cheese

1 garlic clove, minced 1 c. chopped carrots

 3 c. tomatoes

1/4 tsp. dried rosemary

3   oz. grated Romano cheese 1 1/3 c. cottage cheese

Saute onions, garlic, mushrooms, carrots, and peppers until soft. Add tomatoes, parsley, basil, oregano, chili powder, rosemary, and pepper. Simmer 15 minutes. Mix together the 3 cheeses. Starting with sauce, layer with 8 cooked lasagna noodles and cheese in an 8 x 12 inch casserole. Bake at 375 degrees for 30 minutes. Makes 4 servings.

COCONUT CUSTARD PIE

4   eggs

4 tbsp. diet oleo

1 tsp. coconut extract 5 tbsp. flour

8 oz. shredded Jicama sweetener = 1/2 c. sugar 1 3/4 c. water

1   1/2 tsp. vanilla 2/3 c. dry milk

2   slices dry bread Dash of salt

Combine all ingredients in blender, except Jicama. Fold in Jicama and pour into crust lined 10 inch pie pan. Bake at 350 degrees for 40 to 45 minutes.

SUGAR FREE APPLE PIE

4 c. sliced, pared apples (preferably yellow delicious)

1/2 c. unsweetened apple juice concentrate (do not dilute) 1 1/2 tsp. cornstarch or tapioca

1 1/2 tsp. cinnamon or apple pie spice

Mix thickener, concentrate, and spices. Pour over apple slices to coat well. Pour into crust lined pie plate. Top with remaining crust. Bake at 425 degrees about 45 minutes until crust is golden and apples are tender. 8 servings each 220 calories. Exchanges = 1 1/2 fruit, 1 bread, 1/2 fat each serving.

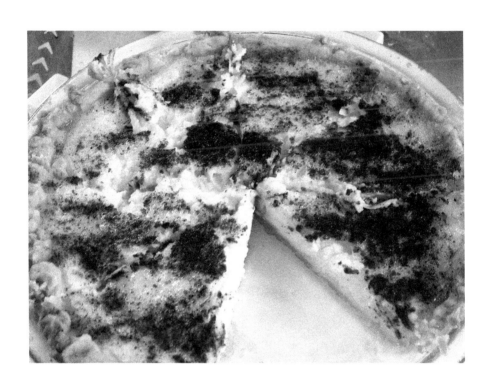

DIABETIC CHEESE CAKE

2/3 c. cottage cheese 1/3 c. cold water

1/2 tsp. vanilla 1/2 c. blueberries 1/3 c. hot water

1/3 c. powdered milk and 3 pkgs. Equal 1 tsp. lemon juice

1   env. unflavored gelatin

Soften gelatin in cold water, then add hot water. Blend until smooth. Add rest of ingredients and blend again until smooth. Stir in blueberries. Chill until firm.

RHUBARB OR CRANBERRY JELLO

2   c. rhubarb

1 pkg. Jello without sugar (raspberry, cherry, or strawberry) 1 1/4 c. water

Put rhubarb in saucepan with 1 cup water. Boil until fruit is soft. Add 1 package of Jello and stir until dissolved. Add 1/4 cup cold water. Stir and pour into individual dishes or a 1 1/2 quart casserole. Chill until set. Cranberries can be used in place of rhubarb.

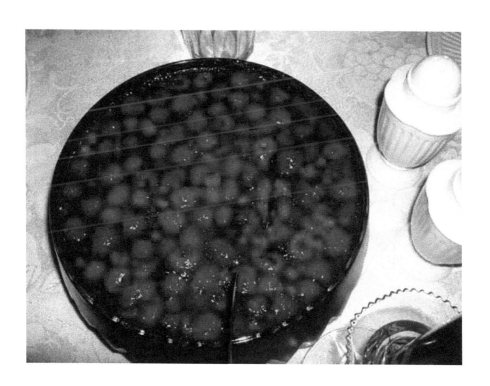

POPSICLES

1 (4 serving size) env. sugar free gelatin

1 (2 qt.) env. sugar free artificially sweetened powdered drink mix (Kool Aid)

In a 2 quart mixing pitcher, dissolve gelatin in 1 cup hot water. Add drink powder; stir, then add 7 cups cold water. Stir. Pour into popsicle cups with handles; freeze. Flavor Suggestions: Raspberry Lemonade Orange Orange Grape Gelatin: Triple berry Lime Hawaiian pineapple Strawberry Raspberry These pops will not melt easily because of the absence of sugar. 1 (2 ounce) popsicle = 2 to 3 calories. 5 to 6 may be eaten per day and is considered a "free" food.

PHUDGESICLES

1 (4 serving size) box sugar free instant pudding (favorite flavor) 3 c. reconstituted non fat dry milk

Whip all together according to directions on pudding package. Pour into popsicle cups with handles; freeze. 1 (2 ounce) pop = approximately 20 calories. 1 per day = "free"*. *"Free" 20 calories or fewer and is not necessary to figure into a diabetic meal plan if limited to one "free" per day.

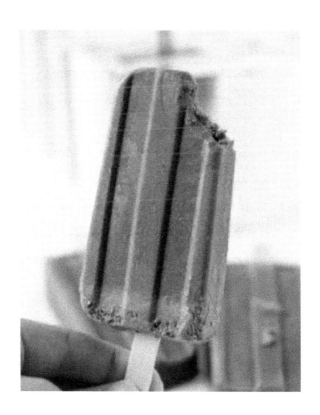

DIABETIC APPLESAUCE COOKIES

1 3/4 c. cake flour 1/2 tsp. salt

1 tsp. cinnamon 1/2 tsp. nutmeg 1/2 tsp. cloves 1 tsp. soda

1/2 c. butter 1 tbsp. sucaryl

1 egg

1 c. applesauce (unsweetened) 1/2 c. All Bran cereal

1/2 c. raisins

Mix together the flour, salt, cinnamon, nutmeg, cloves, and soda.
Mix together butter, sucaryl, and egg until light and fluffy. Add flour
mixture and applesauce alternately, mixing well after each addition.
Fold in raisins and All Bran. Drop on greased cookie sheet. Heat
oven to 375 degrees. Bake for 20 minutes or until golden brown.

DIABETIC SPICE OATMEAL COOKIES

1   c. water

2   c. raisins

4 tbsp sweetner

½ c butter

½ tsp salt

¼ tsp allspice

½ tsp cinnamon

1 tsp soda

1/8 tsp nutmeg 2 ½ c oatmeal

½ c chopped nuts

Boil water and raisins. Cool for 5 minutes. Add all the other ingredients. Form into balls and bake on lightly greased cookie sheet for 15 minutes at 325 degrees.

DIABETIC COOKIES

1 3/4 c. flour

1 tsp. cinnamon 1/2 tsp. nutmeg 1/2 tsp. cloves

1 tsp. baking soda 1/2 c. margarine 1/2 c. Sugar Twin 1 egg

1 c. unsweetened applesauce 1/2 c. raisins, chopped

1 c. All Bran Buds

1/2 c. finely chopped nuts

Preheat oven to 350 degrees. Sift together flour, cinnamon, nutmeg, cloves and baking soda. In large bowl, mix together margarine, artificial sweetener and egg. Mix in dry ingredients, alternating with applesauce. Fold in bran, raisins and nuts and mix thoroughly. Drop onto greased cookie sheet by tablespoons. Lightly flatten with fork, dipped in milk. Bake for 7 8 minutes.

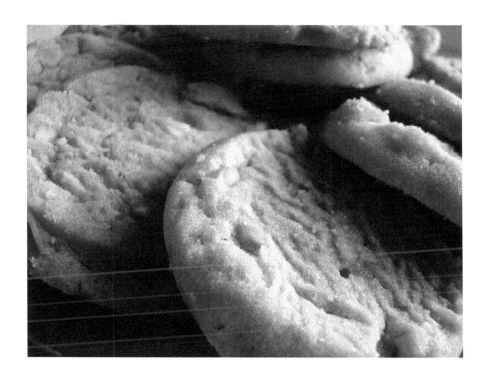

DIABETIC PUMPKIN PIE

1 sm. pkg. sugar free vanilla pudding 1 1/2 c. milk (whole or nonfat)
1 c. canned pumpkin 1/4 tsp. cinnamon 1/4 tsp. nutmeg
Artificial sweetener to equal 1 tsp. sugar 1 baked 8 inch pie crust

Place pudding mix in a saucepan. Gradually add milk. Cook and stir over medium heat until mixture comes to a boil. Remove from heat and add pumpkin, spices and sweetener; mix well. Pour into baked crust. Chill until firm, about 3 hours.

DIABETIC WHIPPED CREAM

1/3 c. instant nonfat dry milk 1/3 c. ice water

1/2 tsp. liquid sweetener

Chill small glass bowl and beaters. Combine ingredients and whip on high speed with mixer until consistency of whipped cream. Makes about 10 servings of 2 tablespoons.

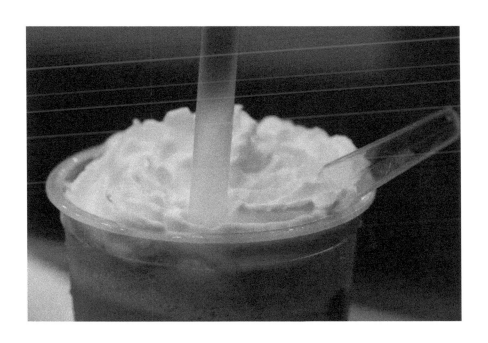

DIABETIC PUMPKIN PIE

1 (16 oz.) can pumpkin

1   (13 oz.) can evaporated milk

2   eggs

1/4 c. Brown Sugar Twin 1/4 c. Sugar Twin

1 tsp. cinnamon 1/2 tsp. salt 1/2 tsp. nutmeg 1/4 tsp. ginger

Sesame Seed Crust

Combine all ingredients and mix well in blender. Pour into Sesame Seed Crust. Bake at 425 degrees for 15 minutes, then reduce heat to 350 degrees, and bake 35 minutes longer. Exchange per serving: 1 bread, 1/2 milk, 1 fat.

 SESAME SEED CRUST

1   c. all purpose flour 1/4 c. sesame seed 1/2 tsp. salt

1/2 c. plus 2 tbsp. corn oil margarine 2 or 3 tbsp. cold orange juice

Combine to make 1 (9 inch) pie shell.

DIABETIC CAKE

2   c. water

2 c. raisins

1   c. unsweetened applesauce 2 eggs

2   tbsp. liquid artificial sweetener 3/4 c. cooking oil

1 tsp. baking soda 2 c. flour

1 1/2 tsp. cinnamon 1/2 tsp. nutmeg

1 tsp. vanilla

Preheat oven to 350 degrees. Cook raisins in water until water evaporates. Add applesauce, eggs, sweetener, cooking oil and mix well. Blend in baking soda and flour. Add cinnamon, nutmeg and vanilla and mix. Pour into greased 8x8 inch cake pan and bake approximately 25 minutes or until done.

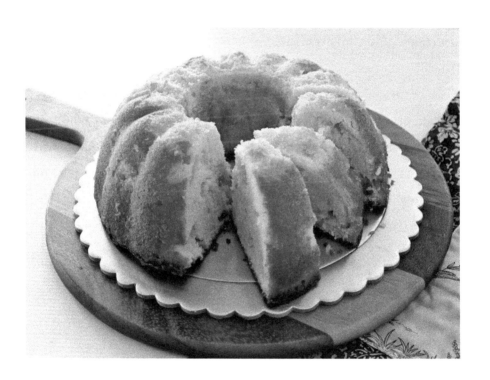

STRAWBERRY PIE
(NO SUGAR)

1 baked pie shell 1 qt. strawberries

3 tbsp. cornstarch

1 (8 oz.) pkg. cream cheese

1 c. apple juice, unsweetened

Slice berries, simmer 1 cup in 2/3 cups apple juice 3 minutes. Mix cornstarch with 1/3 cup apple juice, stir in berries. Stir constantly 1 minute until thick. Spread softened cheese over pie crust, put berries on cheese, pour cooked berries on top. Garnish with whipped cream and a few berries. Chill 3 to 4 hours.

SUGAR-FREE APPLE PIE

4 c. sliced peeled apples

1/2 c. undiluted frozen apple juice concentrate 1 1/2 to 2 tsp. tapioca, cornstarch or flour

1/2 tsp. lemon juice (optional)

1/2 to 1 tsp. cinnamon, nutmeg or apple pie spice

Divide pastry into 2 parts and roll thin to fit an 8 or 9 inch plate. Set aside. Mix apples, apple juice concentrate, thickener and spice and stir until apples are well coated. Add lemon juice, if desired, to keep apples lighter colored. Taste 1 piece of apple to check the spice. Pour into the pastry lined pie pan and top with the second crust or pastry strips. Seal the edges and cut slits in the top crust to allow steam to escape. Bake at 425 degrees for 40 45 minutes until golden brown. Serve warm or cold. NOTE: Apples have some natural pectin, but a small amount of thickener is necessary to hold the sweet concentrate of the apples for an even flavor. One serving (including the crust)-- 220 calories; 1 1/2 fruit exchanges; 1 bread exchange; 1 fat exchange.

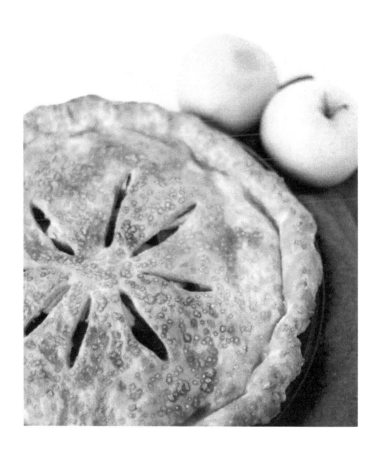

APPLE PIE
(NO SUGAR)

4 c. apple

1/2 c. frozen apple juice concentrate, undiluted 2 tsp. tapioca or cornstarch

1/2 to 1 tsp. cinnamon

Mix apples and all ingredients until well coated; pour into pastry shell and top with pastry. Bake at 425 degrees for 40 to 45 minutes.

POLISH SAUSAGE STEW

1 can cream of celery soup 1/4 c. brown sugar

27 oz. can sauerkraut, drained

1 1/2 lb. polish sausage, cut in 2 inch pieces 4 med. potatoes, pared and cubed

1 c. chopped onion

4 oz. shredded Monterey Jack cheese

Cook sausage,potatoes, and onion until done. Mix soup, sugar & sauerkraut, cook until blended. Mix with other ingredients and top with cheese.

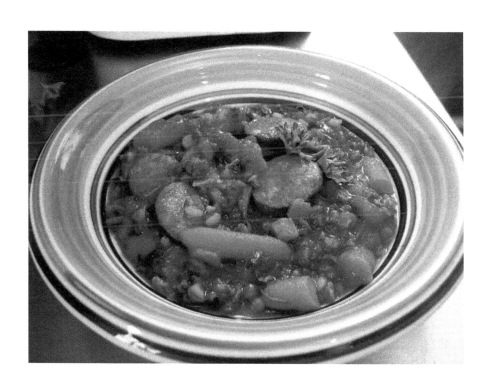

KRAUTRUNZA

1 link (approximately 1/4 lb.) German sausage 1 lb. ground beef

1 sm. head cabbage 1 med. onion

Salt and pepper Yeast dough

Brown meats and add other ingredients, cook until tender. serve

GERMAN SAUERKRAUT

1 can Bavarian sauerkraut, partially drained 1 apple, cored and sliced

1   onion, chopped

2   or 3 slices bacon

Mix together and cook until all is tender.

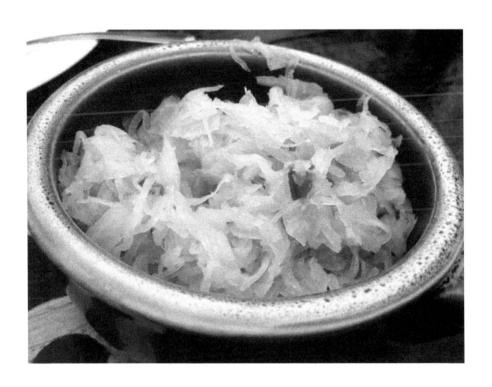

POLISH BIGOS AND KLUSKI

2 lb. ground beef 3 tbsp. Crisco

2 c. diced green pepper 2 c. sliced onions

10 1/2 oz. can tomato soup #2 can tomatoes

3/4 c. water

1 2 tbsp. salt

1/4 tsp. black pepper

1/8 tsp. red pepper (optional) 1/2 pkg. kluski noodles

Brown ground beef. Then add peppers, onions, cook until lightly sauteed. Cook noodles per package direction. Add the rest of the ingredients and cook until well blended. Mix sauce with noodles or let them put on their own sauce.

PATCHLINGS

5 c. flour

1 egg

1 tbsp. shortening

1 c. milk

Mix all ingredients together, drop on cookie sheet, and bake at 350 degrees for about 10 min.

WALNUT DREAMS

¼ lb margarine

1   ½ c. + 1 tbsp brown sugar 1 ½ c. chopped walnuts

2   eggs (beaten)

1 ½ tsp baking powder 1 tsp vanilla

½ c. coconut

Mix all ingredients together and blend thoroughly. Drop on cookie sheet , bake at 325 degrees until lightly brown.

SUGAR-FREE CHERRY OATS MUFFIN

1 1/4 cups unbleached flour

1   1/4 teaspoons baking powder 3/4 teaspoon baking soda

1/4 teaspoon lite (or regular) salt 2/3 cup all fruit black cherry jam

1/3 cup apple juice concentrate 1/2 cup cherry juice concentrate

2   1/2 to 3 Tablespoons canola or safflower oil 1/4 cup water

2 egg whites or 1/3 cup egg white product 1 1/2 cups thin rolled (quick) oats

Preheat your oven to 350 degrees.Sift dry ingredients together and set aside. In a different bowl, lightly beat egg whites or eggbeaterss, and mix in all wet ingredients. Mix liquid and dry ingredients,with a fork, just enough to moisten. Next, gently fold in oats and mix well.

Fill muffin tins 3/4 full, and bake at 350 degrees for 18 to 25 minutes. Check for doneness with a toothpick, if it comes out clean, they're done. Cool about 10 15 minutes. Serve warm or at room temperature. Makes 12 muffins

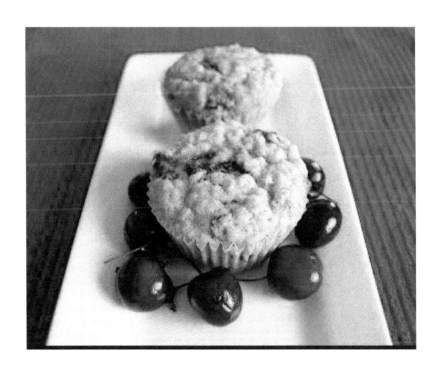

MOM'S WIENER SOUP

4 wieners

1 onion

1 qt. milk

1   1/2 tsp. salt 4 tbsp. butter

2   tbsp. flour

2 c. cooked, diced potatoes 1/4 tsp. pepper

Brown potatoes, wieners and onions in 2tbsp butter. Mix milk, salt, pepper, flour and other 2 tbsp butter together, stir constantly until mixture boils and becomes smooth. Then mix everything together in a soup pan or pot, cook until everything is hot, then serve.

GRANDMA LOE'S SKILLET CAKE

1 3/4 c. cake flour

1 tsp. baking powder 1/4 tsp. soda

1/4 tsp. salt 1 c. sugar

1/4 c. melted margarine 1 egg

1 tsp. vanilla Buttermilk

Put margarine in cup, add egg and fill cup with buttermilk. (Blend with dry ingredients.) (beat) Before last line sift flour, baking powder, soda, salt and sugar into bowl. Then beat with first mixture. Pour into skillet and top with topping.

TUITTI FRUITTI TOPPING

1 c. drained fruit cocktail 1/2 c. brown sugar

1/4 c. chopped walnuts 1/4 c. margarine

Spoon fruit cocktail over top of batter, sprinkle brown sugar and walnuts on top of fruit cocktail, then drizzle with melted margarine

ALMOND PRUNE TOPPING

1 c. cooked prunes, halved 1/2 c. brown sugar

1/4 c. slivered almonds 1/4 c. margarine

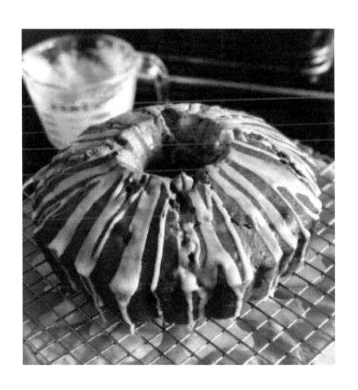

MOM'S BEEF STEW

1/4 c. ginger ale

1 tbsp. red wine vinegar 1 can consomme soup Salt and pepper

1/4 c. flour

1 lb. lean stew meat

1/4 lb. mushrooms, sliced 2 med. potatoes, cut up 2 carrots, sliced

1 onion, sliced

Brown stew meat and sautee with onions and mushrooms. Add all ingredients into pot and cook until meat is and vegetables are tender.

IOCOA EGG PANCAKES

8 eggs, whip hard 1 tsp. salt

2 1/2 c. milk or water 1 c. flour

Mix all ingredients and pour onto grill. Cook on each side until lightly brown.

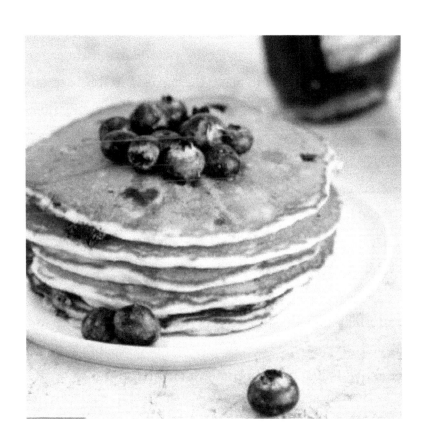

DIABETIC BEEF PASTIES

Crust- 3/4 tsp. Salt 1/4 c. plus
2 tsp. vegetable shortening 1 egg
Water

Put flour and salt in mixing bowl. Cut in shortening. Beat egg in a measuring cup. Add water to make 1/2 cup, add to flour and mix until well moistened. Divide dough into 6 balls. On lightly floured board, roll balls into circles between waxed paper. Then set aside.

FILLING

3/4 lb. coarsely ground beef (raw) 2 c. diced raw potato
3/4 c. diced raw carrot 3/4 c. diced celery
1 tsp. salt
1/4 tsp. black pepper 2 tbsp. water

Once all filling ingredients have been well mixed. Spoon on to dough, and wrap around beef. Bake at 350 degrees for about 10 - 15 min or until dough has become golden brown.

TUNA SUPREME

1 sm. can tuna, water packed 3 hard boiled eggs, diced

1   c. American cheese, diced

2   tbsp. each chopped sweet pickles, mince onion, chopped celery and cut up stuffed olives

1/2 c. mayonnaise or Miracle Whip

Mix all ingredients and serve on bread or lettuce leaf

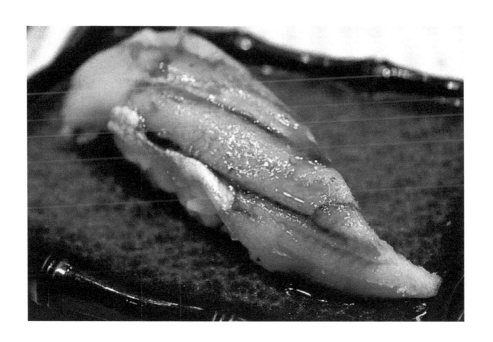

DIABETIC SPICY MEATBALLS

1   lb. lean ground beef 1/2 c. chili sauce

2   tsp. prepared horseradish 1/2 c. minced onion

2 tsp. Worcestershire sauce 1/2 tsp. salt

2 tbsp. corn oil

Mix all ingredients well, roll into balls, and brown in corn oil. Drain on paper towels.

DIABETIC SPICY SAUSAGE

2 lb. extra lean ground pork 2 tsp. crushed dried sage

1 tsp. freshly ground black pepper 1 tsp. fructose

1 tsp. garlic powder 1/2 tsp. onion powder 1/2 tsp. ground mace 1/4

tsp. ground allspice 1/4 tsp. salt

1/8 tsp. ground cloves

Mix all ingredients thourghly. Then make into patties and brown until done.

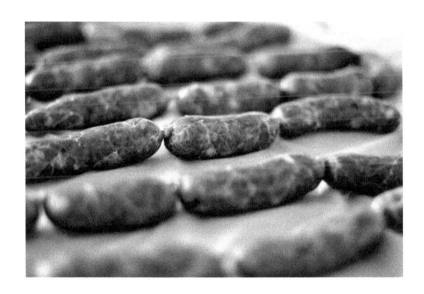

PORK CHOPS & STUFFING

5 pork chops

1   box croutons, prepared to box directions, as stuffing 1/4 c. water

Brown pork chops, make sure cooked well. Serve with stuffing.

DIABETIC APPLESAUCE CAKE

2   c. raisins

2 c. water 3/4 c. oil

4 tbsp. Featherweight sweetener 2 eggs

2 c. flour

1 tsp. soda

1 1/2 tsp. cinnamon 1/2 tsp. nutmeg 1/2 tsp. salt

1/2 c. nuts (if desired)

1   c. unsweetened applesauce

Sift all dry ingredients together and set aside. In a separate bowl mix all wet ingredients. Mix wet and dry ingredients together and mix well, then fold in applesauce, nuts and raisins. Pour in a greased and floured cake pan unless using a non stick pan. Bake at 350 degrees for 25 -30 minutes or until cake springs back when lightly touched in the middle.

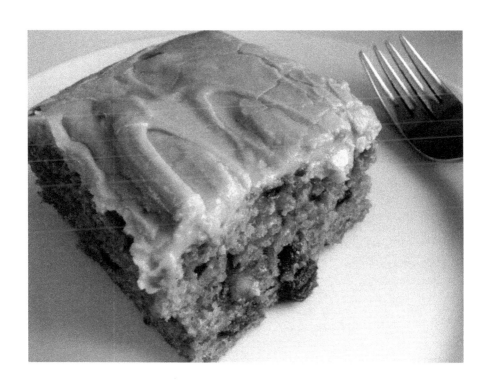

BANANA BREAD

2   c. all purpose flour 1 tsp. baking soda

1 tsp. baking powder

1 1/2 tsp. pumpkin pie spice 2 ripe bananas (mashed)

6 oz. can frozen orange juice 2 eggs

1 c. raisins Nuts (optional)

Sift all dry ingredients together and set aside. In a separate bowl mix all wet ingredients and mashed bananas. Mix wet and dry ingredients together and mix well, then fold in, nuts and raisins. Pour in a greased and floured loaf pan unless using a non stick pan. Bake at 350 375 degrees for 30 45 minutes or when knife comes out clean.

DIABETIC CHOCOLATE CHIP COOKIES

1/2 c. butter

1/3 c. brown Sugar Twin 1 egg

1 1/2 tsp. vanilla extract 1 1/3 c. all purpose flour 2 tsp. baking powder 1/2 tsp. baking soda 1/2 tsp. salt

 3/4 c. skim milk

1/2 c. semi sweet chocolate chips

Cream butter, brown sugar twin, vanilla and egg together. Sift all dry ingredients together in a separate bowl. Add milk, dry ingredients and chocolate chips to creamed mixture. Drop onto cookie sheet. Bake at 325 350 degrees for 7 10 min. or until lightly brown.

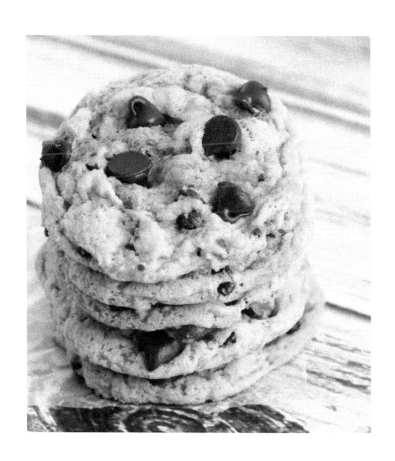

WACHY CHOCOLATE CAKE

1   1/2 c. cake flour 1/4 c. cocoa

2   tbsp. granulated sugar replacement 1 tsp. baking soda

1/2 tsp. salt 1 c. water

1 tbsp. white vinegar

1/4 c. safflower or corn oil 1 tsp. vanilla extract

1 egg

Sift all dry ingredients together and set aside. In a separate bowl mix all wet ingredients. Mix wet and dry ingredients together and mix well. Pour in a greased and floured cake pan unless using a non stick pan. Bake at 350 degrees for 25 -30 minutes or until cake springs back when lightly touched in the middle.

APPLE PIE, SUGARLESS

12 oz. can concentrated apple juice 3 tbsp. cornstarch

1 tsp. ground cinnamon 1/8 tsp. salt

9 inch unbaked pie shell

5 sweet tasting apples, sliced

Mix all ingredients and bring to a boil. When mixture starts to thicken remove from heat. Pour into pie crust. Bake at 350 375 degrees or until golden brown.

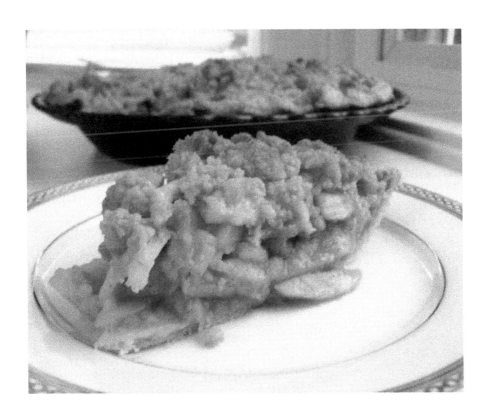

APPLESAUCE COOKIES

1/2 c. all purpose flour 1 tsp. ground cinnamon 1/2 tsp. baking soda

1/4 tsp. allspice

1/2 c. quick rolled oats 1/2 c. raisins Nutmeats (Optional)

1/2 c. unsweetened applesauce 1 egg, beaten

1/4 c. shortening

2 tsp. vanilla extract

1/4 tsp. orange flavoring (optional)

Sift all dry ingredients (including oats) together in a separate bowl. In a separate bowl mix applesauce, eggs, vanilla, orange flavoring (optional) dry ingredients and nuts. Drop onto cookie sheet. Bake at 325 350 degrees for 7 10 min. or until lightly brown.

DIABETIC OATMEAL COOKIES

3/4 c. vegetable shortening 1/2 c. Brown Sugar Twin 1/2 c. white Sugar Twin

1 egg

1/4 c. water

1 tsp. vanilla extract 1 c. all purpose flour 1 tsp. salt

1/2 tsp. baking soda 1 c. raisins

3 c. rolled oats, quick cooking or regular

Cream shortening,sugars, vanilla and egg together. Sift all dry ingredients together in a separate bowl. Add water, dry ingredients, raisins and oats to creamed mixture. Drop onto cookie sheet. Bake at 325 350 degrees for 7 10 min. or until lightly brown

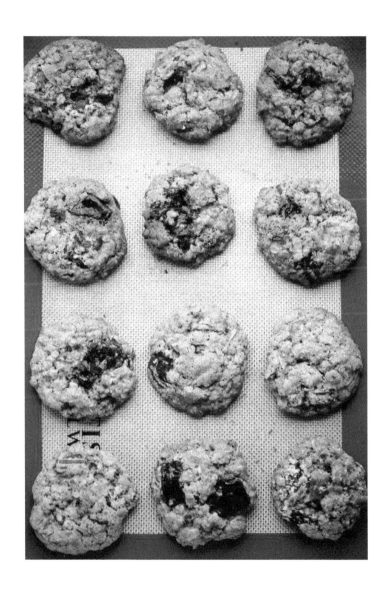

9 781802 748413